# The Injured Hand

H. R. MITTELBACH

# The Injured Hand

## A Clinical Handbook for General Surgeons

*Includes 210 illustrations*

*Translated by Terry Telger*

**Springer-Verlag**
*New York    Heidelberg    Berlin*

**H. R. Mittelbach, M.D.**
*Chefarzt der chirurg. Abteilung*
  *des Städtischen Krankenhauses*
*6780 Pirmasens*
*West Germany*

**Library of Congress Cataloging in Publication Data**

Mittelbach, Hans Reiner.
  The injured hand.

  Translation of Die verletzte Hand.
  Includes index.
  1.   Hand—Wounds and injuries.   2.   Hand—
Surgery.   I.   Title.   [DNLM:   1.   Hand injuries.
WE830  M682v]
RD559.M5713          617′.575          79-219

Title of the German Original Edition: *Die verletzte Hand.* Springer-Verlag
Berlin   Heidelberg   New York, 1977.

Printed in the United States of America.

The use of general descriptive names, trade names, trademarks, etc., in this
publication, even if the former are not especially identified, is not to be taken as
a sign that such names, as understood by the Trade Marks and Merchandise
Marks Act, may accordingly be used freely by anyone.

9  8  7  6  5  4  3  2  1

ISBN 0-387-**90365**-8  Springer-Verlag   New York  Heidelberg   Berlin
ISBN 3-540-**90365**-8  Springer-Verlag   Berlin  Heidelberg   New York

# Foreword

A specialist in hand surgery will not be available at all hospitals for some years. In the meantime, the fate of the patient will continue to rest in the hands of the surgeon who first treats him. It is essential, therefore, that both the novice and the accomplished surgeon have a sound grasp of the diagnostic and therapeutic fundamentals of hand surgery.

The material in this book is presented in a clear, practical manner by a general surgeon who has successfully practiced hand surgery; the result is an especially useful and rewarding book. Many acute situations in hand surgery are not as complicated as they appear to be, whereas other problems can be handled only after much study and experience.

Based on his experience with over 7000 general and emergency operations yearly at the Ludwigshafen Surgical Clinic and after years of intensive work in the field of hand surgery, my medical chief, Dr. H. R. Mittelbach, has taken the time and trouble to write this handbook for general and clinical practice. For the practicing surgeon and especially the resident, the most important aspects of the treatment of hand injuries have been presented in a clear, concise manner. The didactic excellence of the material, its novel format, and the simple yet forceful drawings that obviate lengthy text descriptions enable the reader to become quickly oriented.

However, the book is more than just a "cookbook" for quick reference. It also provides instructive reading for the general surgeon who wishes to become more familiar with the subject of hand surgery. Overly specialized material has been purposely omitted. Based on my own experience in the clinic and in the classroom, I believe that this book will be an excellent guide for the general surgeon.

*Heinz Gelbke*

# Preface

Marc Iselin wrote that a shattered hand or a very serious hand injury is no longer in the province of the general surgeon, who, especially in his early years, lacks the knowledge necessary to assess the eventual consequences. One is tempted to agree with this assertion when one realizes that the young surgeon on night duty, who can generally handle problems in abdominal surgery, may be hard pressed to deal with even minor hand injuries. This is more a problem of inadequate or half-hearted training than a lack of interest, inasmuch as the treatment of hand injuries continues to be regarded as "minor surgery." Hence the call for the specialist, and rightly so. However, it is doubtful whether the specialist alone is capable of solving the problem of hand surgery, since for organizational and personal reasons most fresh hand injuries will continue to come before the general surgeon and his assistants. Even Iselin concedes that it would be better for the time being to teach the general surgeon what hand surgery is than to train hand specialists "who are motivated by an inner call and external circumstances" and who, one might add, will then wish to earn a living.

Thus, the young surgeon must learn how to examine a hand injury correctly and thoroughly. In view of the complex structure of the hand, this is no easy task. He must master many techniques for the care of each anatomical substrate and must know what treatment to administer immediately and what can be deferred. He must recognize the possibilities of subsequent reconstructive surgery, which is best left to the specialist, and must therefore preserve important structures during primary treatment. At the same time, he should recognize what structures must be sacrificed so as not to jeopardize remaining functions. He must have the courage and imagination to cope successfully with novel situations. He must understand that, where the hand is concerned, function ranks above appearance, and he must learn to recognize his own limits. It will quickly become apparent that such skills cannot be acquired without a profound knowledge of general surgery.

It is to these points that this book is addressed. It is based on my 20-year experience as a general surgeon with a career-long interest in hand surgery. It is therefore written primarily for the young surgeon who is confronted with hand injuries that he may or may not be prepared to deal with. He would do well to have this book readily available during night duty for reference. Thanks are due to the publisher for recognizing his needs.

The "specialist," on the other hand, can lay this book aside. It will teach him nothing new, and he is likely to find it incomplete. This statement is based largely on the fact that, at present, as continual progress is made in the field of hand surgery and there is a general trend toward the increased operative treatment of injuries, conservative and simple operative (and thus lower risk) forms of treatment are unjustly threatened with extinction.

This book may be regarded as a reference book that covers only those procedures and techniques that my own experience with hand surgery has shown to be practicable even by less experienced surgeons. For didactic reasons, the basic rules of hand surgery have been repeated where they apply. Bibliographic citations have been purposely held to a minimum, but they are sufficient to enable the interested reader to pursue a given subject. More exhaustive information can be obtained from the *Bibliography of Surgery of the Hand* published by the American Society for Surgery of the Hand.

The fact that this book is already in its third printing in Germany and the reports that it has enabled even younger assistants to acquire a remarkable feel for difficult procedures in the operating room have confirmed the concept behind this book.

I wish to express my thanks to my first teacher, Professor Hilgenfeldt of Bochum, the pioneer of hand surgery in the German-speaking world, who taught me the principles of hand surgery within the context of general surgery, and to Professor Gelbke of Ludwigshafen/Rhein, who gave me ample opportunity to turn these principles into reality at a large general surgical clinic where accident surgery and reconstructive surgery are still routinely practiced.

*H. R. Mittelbach*

# Contents

# Functional Anatomy and Diagnostics in Hand Surgery

In hand surgery, as in general surgery, diagnosis precedes treatment. This fact is often forgotten. The relatively simple access to the numerous densely arranged, functionally important structures tempts one to postpone the diagnosis of fresh open injuries until the operative phase of the treatment, at which time the appropriate measures are taken "according to the conditions found." Closed injuries are frequently dismissed as trivial by a glance at an unremarkable x-ray. This practice needlessly jeopardizes the function of the hand, which cannot always be restored even by costly and time-consuming reconstructive measures.

Hand surgery only *appears* to be "minor surgery," otherwise there would be no hand specialists. However, because most hand injuries are, and will continue to be, treated initially by nonspecialists—a fact which is unchanged by the "delayed operation" concept to be discussed later— every practitioner of surgery should recall the important morphological details of the hand *before* treating the hand injury and should not hesitate to refer to an anatomical atlas in order to arrive at an accurate preoperative diagnosis. Only in this way can grave errors be avoided. A thorough knowledge of hand morphology is essential. Why else does the phrase "injury of the superficial extensor tendon of the index finger" appear again and again in examination reports, and why are nerve lesions or closed ligament injuries so often overlooked?

The knowledge of hand morphology is not enough, however, for the successful practice of hand surgery. Equally important is an understanding of the interaction of the various morphological structures and the function of the human hand as an organ of grasp and touch.

## I. Functional Anatomy of the Hand

The coordination of its supportive and motor functions with its sensory functions makes the hand an organ of grasp and touch. All the posi-

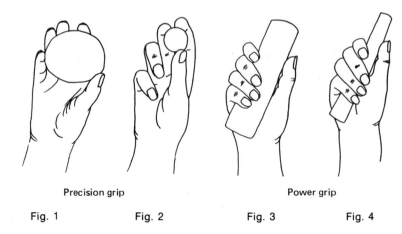

Precision grip                Power grip

Fig. 1           Fig. 2           Fig. 3           Fig. 4

tions that the hand assumes in grasping an object derive from two basic forms: the precision grip and the power grip (Napier) (Figures 1–4).

The *precision grip* grasps an object between the flexor surfaces, generally the bulbs of the fingers, with the long fingers in opposition to the thumb and a counterpressure provided by abduction. The wrist joint is stabilized in moderate expansion. The number of long fingers involved depends on the size of the object. The thumb plays an essential role in this grip.

In the *power grip* the object is held only by the partially flexed long fingers. The thumb and thenar eminence lie more or less adducted in the volar plane and control the direction in which the force is exerted. The wrist is fixed in the intermediate position with a slight inclination toward the ulnar side.

For the precision grip to be executed properly, sensation is essential for all the digits involved. In the power grip, sensation is needed at least in the thumb, which acts as the controlling element. Neither grip can be executed without participation of the thumb. We can thus appreciate the central importance of the opposable thumb in surgery of the hand.

Zur Verth has devised a more practical system for classifying grips according to four primary forms: the pinch grip, key grip, gross grip, and hook grip (Figures 5–8).

This system is useful in describing remaining functions or functions restored by reconstructive surgery and thus tells us something about the functional value of the hand.

## A. Supportive and Motor Apparatus

If we consider Napier's basic forms of grasp, we see that three more or less mobile elements of the hand (namely, the thumb and first metacar-

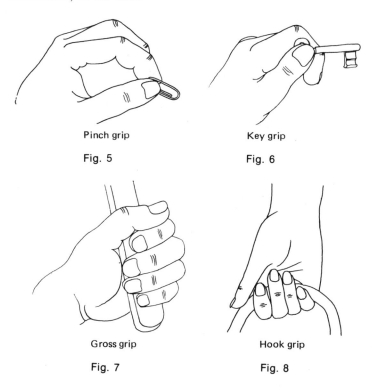

Pinch grip

Fig. 5

Key grip

Fig. 6

Gross grip

Fig. 7

Hook grip

Fig. 8

pal, the index finger, and the functionally linked third through fifth fingers with the fourth and fifth metacarpals) are grouped about a central fixed unit comprised of the distal row of carpal bones and the second and third metacarpals (Figure 9).

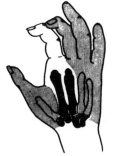

Fig. 9

## 1. Fixed Central Unit of the Supportive Apparatus

The skeletal members of this unit (the distal row of carpal bones and the second and third metacarpals) possess only a small range of movement due to the presence of tight ligaments. The entire unit is moved or fixed as needed by the major wrist muscles inserted into the second and third metacarpals (the radial flexor and the short radial extensor of the wrist) and thus serves as the operating base for the mobile parts of the hand.

The carpal bones form the transverse carpal arch, which is held together by the transverse carpal ligament. From this arch the longitudinal arch of the hand arises, which includes the phalanges via the second and third metacarpals.

Opposing the static transverse carpal arch is the dynamic transverse metacarpal arch, which is formed when the thenar muscles supplied by the median nerve and the hypothenar muscles supplied by the ulnar nerve contract and, owing to the loose fourth and fifth carpometacarpal joints and the transverse capitular ligaments, produce an approximation of the thumb and hypothenar.

2. Dynamic Elements of the Supportive Apparatus

a. *Thumb Ray*

Nine muscles, five short and four long, enable the thumb to exercise its central function during grasping:

| *Short Muscles of the Thumb* | *Long Muscles of the Thumb* |
|---|---|
| First dorsal interosseous | Long extensor |
| Adductor | Short extensor |
| Short abductor | Long abductor |
| Short flexor | Long flexor |
| Opposing | |

The thumb ray owes its high mobility to the saddle joint, which allows it to swivel from adduction to full opposition, the most important motors being the opposing muscle, the superficial head of the short flexor of the thumb, and the short abductor of the thumb. These muscles are supplied by the median nerve, while the remaining short muscles of the thumb are supplied by the ulnar nerve.

b. *Index Finger*

The index finger plays the most important interactive role with the thumb owing to the relative independence of its movements by three short and four long muscles.

c. *Third through Fifth Fingers and Fourth*
   *and Fifth Metacarpals*

Owing to the hypothenar muscles (short flexor of the little finger, abductor, and opposing), these elements form the true opponent of the thumb in the gross grip. The activity of the long fingers is controlled by the long extensors (common extensor of the fingers and the second and fifth extensor proprius) and flexors (superficial and deep flexors), as well as by the short interosseous and lumbrical muscles. The common extensor of the fingers and third through fifth deep flexor muscles can act only in common, because their tendons arise from muscle bellies which are continuous. The remaining muscles give the associated finger a certain degree of independent motion.

When we speak of extensors and flexors, we must realize that these seemingly clearly defined anatomical terms assume a somewhat different aspect within the context of the functional anatomy of the hand:

The wrist flexors, finger extensors, and finger abductors are synergists.
The wrist extensors, finger flexors, and finger adductors are synergists.
The interosseous and lumbrical muscles act both as finger flexors (basal joint) and finger extensors (middle and terminal joints).

## 3. Joints

The numerous and varied positions that the hand skeleton must assume in order to fulfill the requirements of prehension are made possible by its high degree of articulation. The radiocarpal joint, in which the first row of carpal bones articulates with the lower end of the radius, where it joins with the ulna via a fibrocartilage pad, contains an additional clearance for articular motion. The relatively loose ligamentous connections between the scaphoid, lunate, and triquetrum, which allow a certain intrinsic mobility, and the mobility of the fourth and fifth carpometacarpal joints are opposed by the rigid block created by the fixed central unit of the supportive apparatus.

Of special importance is the first carpometacarpal joint, a saddle joint which, owing to its great freedom of motion, is the "key joint" of the thumb.

The finger joints, consisting of the metacarpophalangeal (basal) joints and the proximal and distal interphalangeal (middle and terminal) joints, have essentially the same structures. The basal joint is of the condyloid type, and its range of motion is limited by the ligament apparatus. Its collateral ligaments are eccentrically arranged so that they are taut in the flexed position but slightly lax in the extended position. They tend to shorten, therefore, when they are immobilized in this position (Figure 10a–c). In addition to the ligament apparatus, these joints are also stabilized by the interosseous muscles, which can carry out this function with no assistance from the ligaments if necessary.

The middle and terminal joints are of the ginglymoid type. Due to the extremely tight capsular ligament apparatus and the insertion of the lateral ligaments at the center of rotation of the phalangeal heads, these

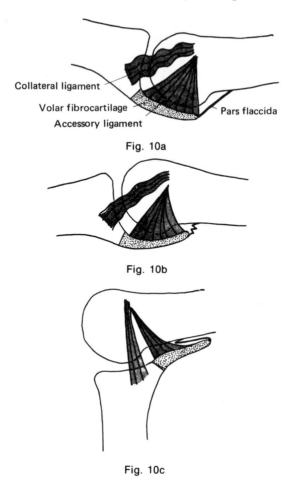

Fig. 10a

Fig. 10b

Fig. 10c

joints are incapable of lateral movement in any position. The volar fibro-cartilage limits the hyperextensibility of all the joints to varying degrees.

## B. Sensation

### 1. Superficial Sensation

Normal cutaneous sensation, or tactile gnosis, with its fine ability to discriminate among different tactile qualities, textures, shapes, and con-sistencies, gives the hand an important place among the sense organs. Only by virtue of its refined sensory qualities is the simple organ of grasp capable of "grasping" in the figurative sense. In terms of sensation, the thumb, index, and middle finger, supplied by the median nerve, are

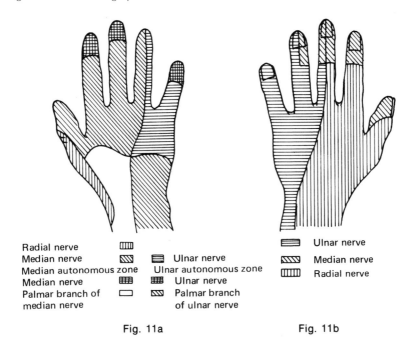

| | | |
|---|---|---|
| Radial nerve | ⬜⬜⬜ | |
| Median nerve | ▨▨ | ▤ Ulnar nerve |
| Median autonomous zone | | Ulnar autonomous zone |
| Median nerve | ⊞⊞⊞ | ⊞⊞ Ulnar nerve |
| Palmar branch of median nerve | ▢ | ▨ Palmar branch of ulnar nerve |

| | |
|---|---|
| ▤ | Ulnar nerve |
| ▨▨ | Median nerve |
| ⬜⬜⬜ | Radial nerve |

Fig. 11a                    Fig. 11b

more important than the ulnar part of the hand, which is supplied by the ulnar nerve. Radial nerve sensation becomes important only if median nerve sensation is lost, at which point secondary forms of grasp are formed with the often remarkably extensive radial-sensory areas on the surface of the thumb and index finger (Figure 11a,b).

## 2. Deep Sensation

Equally important for hand function is deep sensation, which not only signals the position of the joints, but also plays a role in the transmission of organic sensation. Its significance in plastic operations, such as the Hilgenfeldt thumb and Littler-Zrubecky flaps, is also mentioned in passing.

## II. Diagnosis in Hand Surgery

A systematic examination procedure, combined with an accurate knowledge of normal hand topography and functional anatomy, is the best prevention against an inadequate or incorrect diagnosis. It is advantageous for practically all tests to be performed by *one* examiner, with the exception of the x-ray examination and neurological consultation.

> **As a rule, an injury of the hand is not examined, but rather the hand is examined for injuries.**

Precise written documentation of test findings is a medical as well as legal necessity. It is accurate only if made during the examination procedure and supplemented by drawings of amputations, wounds, or scars as well as x-ray films. The use of a dictaphone facilitates these tasks, as does the taking of function photographs.

## A. Procedure for Examining Fresh Injuries

### 1. General History

Metabolic diseases, circulatory disorders, previous accidents, occupation and jobs done at the workplace, and right- or left-handedness are noted.

### 2. Special History

Circumstances of the accident and the accident mechanism are recorded.

### 3. X-ray Examination of the Whole Hand
(Standard Planes)

Bone injuries, dislocations, and pathology unassociated with the accident are looked for.

### 4. Skin and Wound

Cuts, lacerations, crush injuries, depth of wound, skin defects, nature and extent of contamination, and circulatory conditions are noted.

### 5. Tendons

*a. Appearance*
Divisions can be detected even in the resting hand by the abnormal position of a finger relative to adjacent healthy fingers or the uninjured side.

*b. Function*

Simple active flexion and extension of each joint are tested. Suspected dysfunction requires further examination.

---

**Wiggling movements do not demonstrate an intact tendon. Full function is the only proof!**

---

6. Nerves

*a. Fingertip Sensation*

Operative inspection of the nerves is mandatory in all injuries near the nerves. The patient's own statements are often unreliable.

*b. Motor Function*

Tests for motor function are indispensible in injuries of the palm, wrist, and forearm.

*i. Median nerve lesion:* Loss of palmar abduction of the thumb (Figure 12a,b).

*ii. Ulnar nerve lesion:* Loss of ability to adduct the thumb or spread the long fingers (Figure 13a,b).

7. Joint Stability

The test must be done on both hands with the proximal portion of the joint stabilized. Local anesthesia may be required.

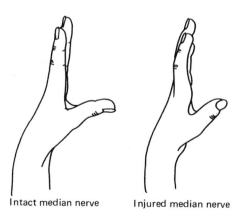

Intact median nerve          Injured median nerve

Fig. 12a                    Fig. 12b

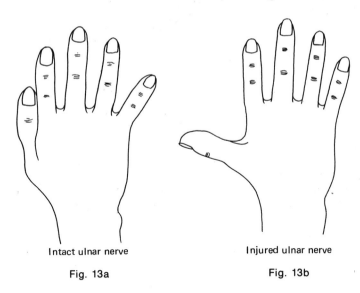

Intact ulnar nerve                    Injured ulnar nerve

Fig. 13a                              Fig. 13b

8. Special X-ray Examinations

Arthrograms with dental film, central carpal films, and laminagrams are obtained.

9. Tissue Vitality

A vital coloration test by dye injection (see chapter on Thermal Injuries) is performed.

B. Examination Procedure for the Preparation of Reconstructive
   Surgery and for Disability Evaluation

All examinations are performed on the whole arm and are compared with findings on the healthy side.

1. General History

2. Special History, Including Prior Treatments and Outcomes

3. Visual Examination

a. Scars

*b. Deformities*

*c. Circulation*

*d. Swelling*

*e. Muscular Atrophy*

*f. Callosity*

*g. Sweat Secretion*

4. Palpation

*a. Test for Tenderness (Repeat with Diversion)*

*b. Test for Painfulness with Passive Movements*

5. Motor Function

Tests of motor function provide information not only on tendon divisions, but also on neuropathy, ischemic contractures, and joint conditions. Scar contractures must be delineated. Record all data!

*a. Techniques for Motor Testing*

*i. Active closure of fist (flexor digitorum superficialis and profundus, deep flexor tendons alone) (Figure 14)*

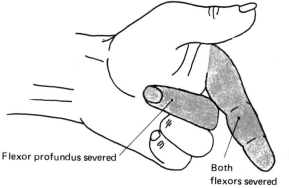

Flexor profundus severed                                  Fig. 14

Both
flexors severed

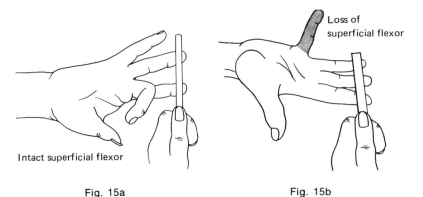

Loss of
superficial flexor

Intact superficial flexor

Fig. 15a                              Fig. 15b

*ii. Flexion of each finger individually, while the remaining fingers are fixed in
extension to eliminate the action of the profundus tendons (superficial flexor tendon alone) (Figure 15a,b)*

*iii. Intrinsic muscle contracture:* The middle and terminal joints can be ac-
tively flexed during flexion of the basal joint; there is no passive flexion
of the middle and terminal joints when the basal joint is fixed in extension.

*iv. Volkmann's contracture:* There is compensation of finger flexion with
increasing flexion of the wrist.

*b. Typical Losses due to Tendon Divisions*

*i. Superficial flexor of the fingers:* There is loss of flexion in the middle
joint (can be tested only if profundus action is eliminated).

*ii. Long flexor of the fingers:* There is loss of flexion in terminal joint.

*iii. Deep and superficial flexors of the fingers:* There is loss of flexion in the
middle and terminal joints (basal joint is flexed by interossei).

*iv. Common extensor of one finger:* There is slight loss of extension in the
basal joint (the tendinous junctures of the adjacent fingers take over a
part of the extension).

*v. Common extensor of several fingers:* There is loss of extension in the
basal joint with free extension in the middle and terminal joints (by interossei and lumbricals).

*vi. Short flexor of the thumb:* There is incomplete flexion of basal joint.

*vii. Long flexor of the thumb:* There is loss of terminal joint flexion.

*viii. Short extensor of the thumb:* There is incomplete extension of the basal joint in some cases.

*ix. Long extensor of the thumb:* The terminal joint extension is absent or weak; the thumb ray cannot be raised above the plane of the other metacarpals.

*x. Short abductor of the thumb:* There is loss of palmar abduction (do not confuse with median nerve paralysis!).

*xi. Long abductor of the thumb:* Fingers cannot be spread in the volar plane (i.e., loss of extension in saddle joint of thumb).

*c. Typical Losses due to Nerve Damage*
Damage may involve disturbances of sensation and trophicity and atrophy of certain muscle groups. Be alert for trick or substitute motions!

*i. Median nerve:* There is loss of full rotation of the thumb ray during opposition or loss of full palmar abduction. "Oath hand" results from high median paralysis.

*ii. Ulnar nerve:* The long fingers cannot be spread or approximated in the volar plane when extended. There is loss of adduction of the thumb extended in the terminal joint. "Claw hand" results from high ulnar paralysis.

*iii. Radial nerve:* There is loss of long finger extension in the basal joints and thumb extension in the terminal joint. "Drop hand" results from high radial paralysis.

*d. Techniques for Testing Sensation*
These tests are very time consuming because slight discrepancies often require multiple follow-up tests. Judgments based on subjective statements by the patient, haphalgesia, or the response to hot and cold are imprecise and therefore unsuitable for surgical purposes.

*i. Two-point discrimination:* The points of a paper clip or caliper are applied to the fingers to determine the smallest interpoint distance at which the patient can still feel two points. The finger tested must be

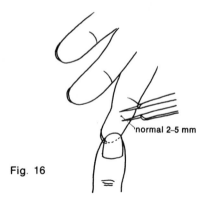

Fig. 16

fixed against the table top to prevent the patient from exerting counter-pressure. The test is begun with a large interpoint distance, which is gradually reduced (Figure 16).

*Normal Values*
| | |
|---|---|
| Fingertip | 2–5 mm |
| Volar surface of proximal phalanx | 6–10 mm |
| Dorsal surface | 12–15 mm |

Tactile gnosis is not present if the two-point discrimination exceeds a distance of 12–15 mm. In this case only protective sensation is still present. Consistent results in 7 of 10 trials are required.

*ii. Picking-up test:* Small objects are picked up with and without benefit of sight. Tactile gnosis is impaired if the patient has difficulty recognizing the objects and shows poor speed and dexterity in picking them up. Watch for trick motions!

*iii. Ninhydrin test (objective sensibility test of Moberg):* When nerve conduction is interrupted, not only tactile gnosis is lost, but also sweat secretion due to the common course of the sympathetic and sensory nerve fibers. Thus, an affected region of the hand is dry in appearance and to the touch.

After the hands are washed to remove traces of sweat from other fingers, the bulbs of the fingers are pressed onto paper strips and the fingers are outlined in pencil. The strip is colored with a 1% solution of ninhydrin in acetone which is acidified with a few drops of acetic acid (shelf life of 2 weeks), and is then developed in an incubator for 3–5 minutes at 110°C. It can later be fixed in a 1% copper nitrate solution in acetone and distilled water in a ratio of 95:5 treated with 5 drops of concentrated nitric acid. This is important for documentation purposes.

Points of sweat secretion appear in the fingerprints as red spots. The presence of neuropathy can be inferred from the number and distribution of the spots (Figure 17).

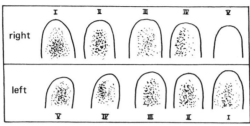

Right ulnar loss

Fig. 17

---

**Some time after the injury, sweat secretion may return, at least in part, without the return of tactile gnosis. The test is therefore only conditionally suited for judging the success of reconstructive surgery.**

---

*e. Typical Causes of Joint Stiffness*

*i. Old nerve injury*

*ii. Tendon adhesions (change in motion range of terminal joints during a positional change of basal joints)*

*iii. Shortening of the lateral ligaments*

*iv. Ischemic contracture*

*f. Circumference Measurements*

Measurements are taken at the following sites: 15 cm above the ulnar condyle; 10 cm below the ulnar condyle with the elbow joint in 90° flexion; the metacarpus (without thumb) above the metacarpal heads; and the elbow joint and wrist joint only in the case of direct joint injury.

*g. Technique for Measuring the Joint*

The rotational movements of the forearm are measured starting from the intermediate (unrotated) position with the elbow joint in 90° flexion and the forearm adjacent to the body. Its deflection is measured in degrees, with the intermediate position representing 0°.

At the wrist joint the angle is measured between the third metacarpal and the ulna and is given in degrees, starting from 0° at the intermediate position.

The finger joints are measured with a small goniometer on the dorsal side. The starting position is full extension, equal to 180°.

The fingertip-to-palm distance is a parameter for the mobility of all three finger joints only if the distance to the transverse volar flexion crease, rather than simply the shortest distance from the fingertips to the hand, is measured.

## 6. X-ray Examination

Standard planes, special projections, and laminagrams are obtained.

**Bibliography**

*Buck-Gramcko, D.:* Objektive Sensibilitätsprüfung. Chir. Plast. Reconstr. 8, 12 (1970).
*Close, R., Kidd, C. C.:* The function of the muscles of the thumb, the index and the long fingers. J. Bone Joint Surg. A.51, 1601 (1969).
*Littler, W. J.:* The physiology and dynamic function of the hand. Surg. Clin. North Am. 40, 259 (1960).
*Lona, Ch.:* Intrinsic–extrinsic muscle control of the hand in power grip and precision handling. J. Bone Joint Surg. A 52, 853 (1970).
*Millesi, H.:* Fermentreaktion und Vitalitätsprüfung. Chir. Plast. Reconstr. 8, 43 (1970).
*Napier, J. R.:* The prehensile movements of the human hand. J. Bone Joint Surg. B 38, 902 (1956).
*Stack, H. G.:* A study of muscle function in the fingers. Ann. R. Coll. Surg. Engl. 33, 307 (1963).
*Tempest, M. N.:* Intravenöse Farbstoffinjektion zur klinischen Beurteilung der Lebensfähigkeit von Gewebe. Chir. Praxis 3, 265 (1961).